MW01122092

To

Mom & Dad
Dunkley

Love
Annemarie

Gary

VEGAN
MEALS FOR A
BETTER
LIFE STYLE

ANNEMARIE GAIRY

authorHOUSE®

AuthorHouse™
1663 Liberty Drive
Bloomington, IN 47403
www.authorhouse.com
Phone: 1-800-839-8640

First published by AuthorHouse 11/15/2011

ISBN: 978-1-4634-3634-6 (e)
ISBN: 978-1-4634-3633-9 (sc)

Library of Congress Control Number: 2011913591

Printed in the United States of America

DEDICATED

This Cook Book is dedicated to my mother Catherine, sister Anjanette and in memory of my Father Roderick Gairy. Over the years their advise (joys and frustrations) with a number of these recipes have refined their frameworks to become what they are. I wish to add mention of my Aunts Irma Morgan and Lema Gairy who have attended several health lecturing sessions In which I have shared in depth rationale as to why these entrees either prevent, improve various diseases and or the degree to which they promote wellness. I would also like to thank my cousin Learie Gairy who challenged me with the idea of arranging this compilation. Special mention and praise is given to Jesus Christ whose inspiration is unfailing and infinitely restorative.

God be merciful unto us and bless us, and cause his face to shine upon us: That thy way may be known upon earth, thy saving health among all nations. Ps 67:1-2

FOREWORD

Meal Preparation is a science. The chemistry of hydrating and or dehydrating different botanical chemicals found in ingredients has the potential to invigorate bodily energy and reduce aging. These natural substances are vitamins, minerals, antioxidants, phytochemicals and chemical constituents which facilitate hormonal activity. It is for this purpose the frameworks outlined in each recipe were done. Christ the creator of such biochemical possibilities designed them to promote physiological, mental and psychological wellness. Hence their increased consumption will yield multiple returns of renewed vigor, and energy.

This Vegan Vegetarian approach to cooking allows for peak nutrient performance, low empty calorie and high Essential fatty acid intake which together may prevent and or improve many Life Style diseases. It is the dietary host that welcomes many health advantages that enhances strength and vigor.

Society is currently attempting to reverse leading risk factors that contribute to obesity, Heart disease and even premature deaths. It is with this understanding healthful strategies have been implemented in each recipe. Each provides a framework reflecting systematic tasty, wholesome entrees to consider as alternatives and then practice with expertise. It is with this endeavour each recipe is shared with you.

Heal me oh Lord and I shall be healed, save me and I shall be Saved, for Thou are my Praise. Jeremiah 17:14

TABLE OF CONTENTS

BREAKFAST ENTREES

ALMOND MILK

BLEND UNTIL SMOOTH:

½ C BLANCHED ALMONDS
1 C HONEY
½ C PEARS (optional)
1 T VANILLA (ALCOHOL FREE)
1t SEA SALT
1C HOT WATER

THEN ADD:
4C WATER AND BLEND, ALMOND MILK WILL REMAIN GOOD IN FRIDGE FOR 1 WEEK. THE ADDITIONAL WATER IS TO PROVIDE FLUID VOLUME ONCE INITIAL INGREDIENTS ARE CREAMED SMOOTHLY IN BLENDER. THIS MILK MAY BE USED IN CEREALS AND FOR BAKING.

OATMEAL MILK

BLEND UNTIL SMOOTH:

1C COOKED OATMEAL
1/2C HONEY
1T VANILLA (ALCOHOL FREE)
1t SEA SALT
½ C OF DRIED DATES
1C HOT WATER

THEN ADD:
4C WATER AND BLEND. (MAY ADD VARIOUS DIRED & OR FRESH FRUIT OF CHOICE IN BLEND) OATMEAL MILK WILL REMAIN GOOD IN FRIDGE FOR 1 WEEK. THE ADDITIONAL WATER IS TO PROVIDE VOLUME ONCE INITIAL INGREDIENTS ARE CREAMED SMOOTHLY IN BLENDER. THIS MILK MAY BE USED IN CEREALS & FOR BAKING.

RICE MILK

BLEND UNTIL SMOOTH:

1C COOKED BROWN RICE
1C HONEY
1T VANILLA (ALCOHOL FREE)
1t SEA SALT
½ C DRIED DATES
1C HOT WATER

THEN ADD:
4C WATER AND BLEND. RICE MILK WILL REMAIN GOOD IN FRIDGE FOR 1 WEEK. THE ADDITIONAL WATER IS TO PROVIDE FLUID VOLUME ONCE INTITIAL INGREDIENTS ARE CREAMED MOOTHLY IN BLENDER. THIS MILK MAY BE USED IN CEREALS AND FOR BAKING.

GRANOLA

2C WATER
12C QUICK OR ROLLED OATS
1C HONEY
1C ALMONDS OR CHOPPED NUTS
2T VANILLA
1C CHOPPED DRIED FRUIT
1T SEA SALT

STIR FIRST FIVE INGREDIENTS . ADD OATS AND NUTS STIRRING ONLY ENOUGH TO MOISTEN OATS. SPREAD UNTO COOKIE SHEETS. BAKE AT 250 F FOR 2 TO 2 ½ HOURS UNTIL DRY. STIRRING EVERY 30-40 MIN. ADD DRIED FRUIT AFTER BAKING.

RICE CEREAL PIE

2C SHORT GRAIN BRON RICE
3T HONEY
1T VANILLA
1t SEA SALT
¼ C-1/2C DRIED FRUIT
4C WATER

RINSE RICE AND ADD REMAINING INGREDIENTS IN
'8x8' PYREX DISH. FILL DISH WITH WATER UP TO RIM.
PLACE LID AND BAKE AT 350 F FOR 2 HOURS.

ALMOND OAT WAFFLE

2 1/2C QUICK / ROLLED OATS
1t SEA SALT
3C WATER
1T VANILLA
3T RAW ALMONDS
3T HONEY
2-3T OF SEASONAL BERRIES OF CHOICE / DRIED FRUIT
OF CHOICE (OPTIONAL)

BLEND SMOOTH ALL INGREDIENTS. POUR INTO HOT
WAFFLE IRON AND BAKE 15-20 MIN EACH.

CASHEW OAT WAFFLE

2 ½ C QUICK / ROLLED OATS
1t SEA SALT
2C SOYMILK
1C WATER
1T VANILLA (ALCOHOL FREE)
3T RAW CASHEWS
3T HONEY

BLEND SMOOTH ALL INGREDIENTS. POUR INTO HOT
WAFFLE IRON AND BAKE 15-20 MIN EACH.

MILLET ALMOND WAFFLE

3C COOKED MILLET
1/2C WATER
1T VANILLA
5T RAW ALMONDS
4T HONEY

BLEND SMOOTH ALL INGREDIENTS. CONSISTENCY OF BATTER MUST BE THICK. POUR INTO HOT WAFFLE IRON AND BAKE FOR 7-10 WITH LID HELD OPEN. THEN COVER WITH LID FOR REMAINING 5-10 MIN. IF LID IS CLOSED TOO SOON THE BATTER WILL LEAK OUT WITH CLOSED LID. THIS IS DUE TO THE FACT THAT BOTH RICE & MILLET ARE GLUTEN FREE GRAINS AND MUST BE BAKED DIFFERENTLY IN WAFFLE IRONS.

BASIC RICE WAFFLE

3C COOKED RICE
1/2 C WATER
1T VANILLA
4 T HONEY

BLEND SMOOTH ALL INGREDIENTS. CONSISTENCY OF BATTER MUST BE THICK. POUR INTO HOT WAFFLE IRON AND BAKE FOR 7-10 WITH LID HELD OPEN. THEN COVER WITH LID FOR REMAINING 5-10 MIN. IF LID CLOSED TOO SOON THE BATTER WILL LEAK OUT WITH CLOSED LID. THIS IS DUE TO THE FACT THAT BOTH RICE & MILLET ARE GLUTEN FREE GRAINS AND MUST BE BAKED DIFFERENTLY IN WAFFLE IRONS.

WHOLE WHEAT BREAD

1C WATER
3C WHOLE WHEAT FLOUR
1/2C OF SOY/RICE MILK
1/2C FLAX SEED (Optional)
1/4C CANOLA OIL
1t YEAST
1-2T HONEY
1t SEA SALT

ALLOW YEAST TO RISE IN LIQUIDS WITH HONEY .
ADD 1C DRY INGREDIENTS AND STIR IN LIQUID FOR
10 MIN. (THIS ALLOWS FOR EVEN SMOOTH TEXTURE
IN BREAD) THEN ADD REMAINING DRY INGREDIENTS
UNTIL MOIST DOUGH. ALLOW DOUGH TO RISE FOR 30
MIN. THEN SHAPE INTO BREAD PANS. ALLOW IT TO
RISE AGAIN FOR 20 MIN. THEN BAKE FOR 50-60 MIN AT
350 F.

WHOLE OAT & WHEAT BREAD

2 C WHOLE WHEAT FLOUR
1C OAT FLOUR
1-1/2C WATER
¼ C CANOLA OIL
1t YEAST
1-2 T HONEY
1t SEA SALT

ALLOW YEAST TO RAISE IN LIQUIDS WITH HONEY. ADD 1C DRY INGREDIENTS AND STIR IN LIQUID FOR 10 MIN. (THIS ALLOWS FOR EVEN SMOOTH TEXTURE IN BREAD) THEN ADD REMAINING DRY INGREDIENTS UNTIL DOUGH IS MOIST. ALLOW DOUGH TO RISE FOR 30 MIN. THEN SHAPE INTO BREAD PANS. ALLOW TO RISE AGAIN FOR 20 MIN. THEN BAKE FOR 50-60 MIN AT 350 F.

DINNER ENTREES

CHICKPEA A LA KING

BLEND

ADD TO SAUCE PAN WITH:

3/4C WATER
2C COOKED CHICK PEAS OR
CAN OF CHICK PEAS (19oz-)
1/2C RAW NUTS/SEEDS OF CHOICE
½ C FROZEN GREEN PEAS
1/4C FLOUR
2/3 C SLICED CARROTS
3T CHICKEN STYLE SEASONING
1t SEA SALT
1/2C CHOPPED ONIONS
1C CHOPPED ONIONS
2 1/4C ADDITIONAL WATER

BLEND SMOOTH FIRST FIVE INGREDIENTS. POUR
INTO SAUCEPAN. RINSE BLENDER WITH ADDITIONAL
WATER AND POUR INTO SAUCE PAN. ADD CHICK PEAS
LIGHTLY BOIL, STIRRING, ABOUT 10-20MIN, UNTIL
THICKENED. ADD VEGETABLES DURING THE LAST 5
MINUTES OF BOILING.

VEGETARIAN CHICKEN STYLE SEASONING

1 1/3C YEAST FLAKES
4T ONION POWDER
3T GARLIC POWDER
3T SEA SALT
1t CELERY SEED
3T ITALIAN SEASONING
2T PARSLEY (DRIED)

BLEND SMOOTH ALL EXCEPT PARSELY. STIR IN PARSLEY. SEAL IN AN AIR TIGHT CONTAINER. MAY USE IN SAME PROPORTIONS AS WHEN USING NON-VEGETARIAN CHICKEN STYLE SEASONING. THE LATER CONTAINS MSG.

RICE & KIDNEY BEANS

3C WATER
1C SOY MILK
2C LONG GRAIN BROWN RICE
1C OF KIDNEY BEANS (KIDNEY STEW OR 1 540ml or 19oz CAN OF KIDNEY BEANS)
3 GARLIC CLOVES
1-2 MEDIUM OMIONS
2T GARLIC, ONION, & PAPRIKA (HUNGARIAN IS HOT TO TASTE) POWDERS
1T SEA SALT
1/8C OF OIL OR 1 CUBE OF COCNUT CREAM

PLACE ALL LIQUIDS AND BEANS IN PYREX DISH. ADD WASHED RICE, GARLIC AND SEASONING POWDERS. SLICE ONIONS AT TOP OF WATER SURFACE AND THEN BAKE AT 350 F FOR 2 HOURS COVERED. ALLOW IT TO BAKE UNCOVERED FOR A FURTHER 10 MIN TO ENHANCE SAVORY TASTE.

RICE AND PIGEON PEAS

3C WATER
1C SOY MILK
2C LONG GRAIN BROWN RICE
1C OF PIGEON PEAS (PIGEON PEAS OR 1 540ml or 19oz
CAN OF PIGEON PEAS)
3 GARLIC CLOVES
1-2 MEDIUM OMIONS
2T GARLIC, ONION, & PAPRIKA (HUNGARIAN IS HOT
TO TASTE) POWDERS
1T SEA SALT
1/8C OF OIL OR 1 CUBE OF COCNUT CREAM

PLACE ALL LIQUIDS AND PEAS IN PYREX DISH. ADD
WASHED RICE, GARLIC AND SEASONING POWDERS.
SLICE ONIONS AT TOP OF WATER SURFACE AND
THEN BAKE AT 350 F FOR 2 HOURS COVERED. ALLOW
IT TO BAKE UNCOVERED FOR A FURTHER 10 MIN TO
ENHANCE SAVORY TASTE.

TASTY RICE

3C WATER
2C LONG GRAIN BROWN RICE
1C SOY MILK
 THREE SLICED GARLIC CLOVES
1/4C VEGETABLE JUICE
1-2 1-2CHOPPED MEDIUM ONIONS
1/8C OF OIL (OF CHOICE)
1T SEA SALT
2T GARLIC, ONION, PAPRIKA (HUNGARIAN TYPE HOT
TO TASTE) POWDERS

PLACE ALL LIQUIDS IN PYREX POT. ADD WASHED RICE,
GARLIC AND SEASONING POWDERS. SLICE ONIONS
AT TOP OF WATER SURFACE LEVEL AND THEN BAKE
AT 350 F FOR 2 HOUR COVERED. ALLOW IT TO BAKE
UNCOVERED FOR A FURTHER A 10;N MIN TO ENHANCE
SAVORY TASTE.

SPINACH CREAM, AVOCADO & RICE

ADD TO POT:

4C WATER
1 PACKAGE OF SPINACH
1 SWEET PEPPER, DICED
3 MEDIUM TOMATOES
1C COCONUT CREAM/MILK
2 LARGE ONIONS
1C OR PACKAGE OF DICED OKRA

WHEN THICKEND ADD:

3T GARLIC POWDER
3T ONION POWDER
3T GARLIC POWDER
1T SEA SALT

BRING TO BOIL INGREDIENTS IN POT THEN ALLOW TO SIMMER OVER A LOW HEAT FOR 1HR. ONCE THICKENED STIR IN SEASONING POWDERS AND COCONUT. ALLOW TO SIMMER FOR ANOTHER 5-10 MIN. THEN BLEND UNTIL SMOOTH IN BLENDER OR WITH USE OF HAND BLENDER IN POT. THIS SPINACH CREAM MAY BE POURED OVER 4-6 CUPS OF PLAIN COOKED OR TASTY RICE PLATE SERVINGS. THIS CREAM MAY BE SERVED OVER PASTA OR BAKED POTATOES AS WELL. *OPTIONAL* CUT CUBBED PIECES OF AVOCADO OVER CREAM ON RICE OR OTHER DISH SERVINGS.

KIDNEY BEAN STEW

6C WATER
2 1/2C DRIED KIDNEY BEANS
3 LARGE ONIONS
5 GARLIC CLOVES
½ C CELERY
1 SWEET PEPPER DICED
1-2T SEA SALT
1T COCONUT CREAM

BRING ALL ITEMS WITH EXCEPTION OF SEA SALT AND COCNUT CREAM TO A BOIL. REDUCE HEAT TO MINIMUM: APPRX '2' ON A STOVE AND ALLOW SIMMERING FOR 1 HOUR. ONCE BEANS HAVE BROKEN OPEN AND WATER HAS DEVELOPED INTO A THICK CREAM. THEN ADD SEA SALT AND COCONUT CREAM.

LENTIL PEAS STEW

6C WATER
2 1/2C DRIED LENTIL PEAS
3 LARGE ONIONS
5 GARLIC CLOVES
½ C CELERY
1 SWEET PEPPER DICED
1 LARGE TOMATOE DICED
1-2T SEA SALT
1T COCONUT CREAM
1C MINT
1C GARLIC CHIVES

BRING ALL ITEMS WITH EXCEPTION OF SEA SALT AND COCNUT CREAM TO A BOIL. REDUCE HEAT TO MINIMUM: APPRX '2' ON A STOVE AND ALLOW SIMMERING FOR 1 HOUR. ONCE PEAS HAVE BROKEN OPEN AND WATER HAS DEVELOPED INTO A THICK CREAM. THEN ADD SEA SALT AND COCONUT CREAM.

ROMANO BEANS STEW

6C WATER
2 1/2C DRIED ROMANO BEANS
3 LARGE ONIONS
5 GARLIC CLOVES
1/2C CELERY
1SWEET PEPPER DICED
2 LARGE TOMOTOES DICED
1C MINT
1-2 SEA SALT

BRING ALL ITEMS WITH EXCEPTION OF SEA SALT TO
A BOIL. REDUCE HEAT TO MINIMUM, APPROX '2' ON
STOVE AND ALLOW BOILING FOR 1 HOUR. ONCE BEANS
HAVE BROKEN OPEN AND WATER HAS DEVELOPED
INTO A THICK CREAM. THEN ADD SEA SALT.

PIGEON PEAS STEW

6C WATER
2 1/2C DRIED PIGEON PEAS
3 LARGE ONIONS
5 GARLIC CLOVES
½ C CELERY
1 SWEET PEPPER DICED
1-2T SEA SALT
2 LARGE TOMATOES DICED
2C CHOPPED SQUASH (OF ANY VARIETY)
1T COCONUT CREAM

BRING ALL ITEMS WITH EXCEPTION OR SEA SALT AND COCNUT CREAM TO A BOIL. REDUCE HEAT TO MINIMUM: APPRX '2' ON A STOVE AND ALLOW SIMMERING FOR 1 HOUR. THEN ADD CHOPPED SQUASH AND ALLOW SIMMERING ONCE PEAS HAVE BROKEN OPEN AND WATER HAS DEVELOPED INTO A THICK CREAM. THEN ADD SEA SALT AND COCONUT CREAM.

CHICK PEA CURRY

SAUTE:

2 TBSP VEGETABLE OIL & 1 LARGE ONION SLICED

THEN ADD:

2 CANS OF CHICK PEAS
1C OF WATER
2 TBSP GARLIC & ONION POWDER
1C CHOPPED PEALED POTATOES
½ C OF VEGETABLE JUICE
2 TBSP TO TUMERIC POWDER
1tsp SEA SALT

SAUTE ONIONS UNTIL FAINTLY BROWN THEN ADD REMAING INGREDIENTS EXCEPT THE TUMERIC TO SIMMER ON A MEDIUM TO LOW STOVE TOP HEAT FOR 1 HOUR. THEN STIR IN TUMERIC & SALT WHERE CURRY SAUCE WILL THICKEN , THUS TURN OFF STOVE WITH CURRY MADE. THIS CURRY MAY BE SERVED WITH RICE & ROTI'S.

LASAGNA
(OR CANTELLONI ROLES)

COLUMN ONE   **COLUMN TWO**

3C PASTA SAUCE   1 PACK OF LASAGNA
2T ONION POWDER   NOODLES
2 MEDIUM SIZE ONIONS SLICED
1T GARLIC POWDER
1 C CHOPPED FIRM TOFU

COLUMN THREE

3C MIXED CUT VEGETABLES OR SPINACH
1T SEA SALT
1 1/3C LENTIL STEW

ALLOW COLUMN ONE TO SIMMER FOR 1HR. WHEN THE PASTA SAUCE THICKENS IT IS READY TO USE FOR LAYERING. PLACE LASAGNA NOODLES IN A CASSAROLE DISH. LAYER LENTIL STEW. SPINACH 1CM THICK, PASTA SAUCE THEN LASAGNA NOODLES. WHEN USING CANTELLONI ROLES FILL ROLES IN THE SAME MANNER WITH INGREDIENTS OF COLUMN THREE.

SPAGHETTI SAUCE CASSEROLE

BOIL FOR 5 MIN:

1 PACK OF WHOLE WHEAT or BROWN RICE SPAGHETTI & or FETTUCINE

LAYER:

SPHAGETTI IN LASAGNA DISH
1CAN OF SHAGETTI/PASTA SAUCE
1CAN OF TOMATO SOUP & OR V8 JUICE
1CAN OF CRISP CORN & OR SWEET PEAS
1C OF CHOPPED CARROTS

POUR CORN, PEAS, CARROTS & THEN SAUCE OVER SPAGHETTI (or FETTUCINE) SPRINKLE 1t SEA SALT OVER INGREDIENTS. THEN BAKE FOR 50 MIN @ 350 F. (ADD SPINACH SAUCE WITH SHAGETTI/PASTA SAUCE IS OPTIONAL FOR BAKING)

SPAGHETTI SOUP CASSEROLE

BOI L FOR 5 MIN:

1 PACK OF WHOLE WHEAT or BROWN RICKE SPAGHETTI
& or FETTUCINE

LAYER:

SPHAGETTI IN LASAGNA DISH

BLEND:

3C SOY MILK
1PACKAGE OF ONIONS SOUP
1TBSP GARLIC POWDER,
2 TBSP ONION POWDER
1tsp SEA SALT
1CAN OF CRISP CORN & OR SWEET PEAS
1C OF CHOPPED CARROTS

SPREAD CORN, PEAS, CARROTS & THEN SOY MILK
BLEND OVER SPAGHETTI (or FETTUCINE). THEN BAKE
FOR 50 MIN @ 350 F

CORN MEAL CASSEROLE

BLEND: ADD:

1CAN CREAMED CORN   1 ¾ CORN MEAL
2 MEDIUM SIZE ONIONS
2T GARLIC POWDER

ADD TO SAUCE PAN:

1C TOMATO SOUP
1 ¼ C COCNUT MILK
1 1/4C SOY/RICE MILK

THEN STIR CORNMEAL IN BLENDED CREAM IN SAUCE
PAN UNTIL THICKENED WITH A MEDIUM TO HIGH
HEAT. CONTINUE TO STIR UNTIL A SMOOTH CREAM
AND TO AVOID CRUSTING OR BURNING AT BOTTOM.
POUR CREAM INTO PYREX DISH(ES) OF CHOICE AND
BAKE FOR 1HR @ 350 F.

CREAMY SCALLOPED POTATOES

BLEND SMOOTH:

3C SOY/RICK MILK
4T ONION POWDER
3T GARLIC POWDER
2T PAPRIKA
¼ C OF NON HYRDROGENATED MARGARINE OR RICE
BUTTER (OPTIONAL)

LAYER:

6-8 LARGE SLICED POTATOES
2-3 LARGE ONIONS

BLEND LIQUID AND SEASONING INGREDIENTS.
PEAL POTATOES AS PREFERED SLICE IN 1/4CM THICK
COOKIE SLICES AND LAYER ONE ROW IN A LASAGNE
DISH. THEN LAYER A ROW OF ¼ CM THICK SLICE OF
ONIONS. THEN POTATOES, FOLLOWED BY ONIONS
UNTIL REACHING LESS THAN ¼ CM OF THE HEIGHT
OF THE DISH. POUR SEASONED LIQUID OVER LAYERED
POTATOES IN DISH. THEN BAKE FOR 50 MIN COVERED,
THEN UNCOVERED FOR 10 MIN @ 350 F.

SHEPPARD'S PIE

BOIL UNTIL SOFT:

5C WATER
8 MEDIUM –LARGE POTATOES

THEN ADD:

½ C SOY/RICE MILK
1C OF NON HYDRGOGENATED MARGARINE OR GRAIN
BUTTERS IN BOOK
2C BEAN/PEA STEW OF CHOICE
1 340ml CAN OF CRISP CORN

ONCE POTATOES ARE SOFT POUR HOT WATER FROM
POT AND ADD SOY MILK & MARGARINE. THEN MASH
UNTIL SMOOTH. LAYER 1/2-1 CM THICK IN CORNING
WARE DISH. THEN SPREAD PRECOOKED BEAN/PEA
FILLING OF CHOICE 1/2-1 CM THICK. FOLLOWED BY
REMAINING PORTION OF MASHED POTATOES. THEN
BAKE @ 350 F FOR 50-60 MIN UNCOVERED.

PASTA STIR FRY

COLUMN ONE

1C VEGETABLE OIL
2 MEDIUM ONIONS SLICED
2CLOVES OF GARLIC
2CLOVES OF GARLIC

COLUMN TWO

1C MIXED
VEGETABLES
3C SLICED CABBAGE
2C SPINACH/SWISS
CHARD
1C V8 VEGETABLE
JUICE

COLUMN THREE:

1 1/2C WHOLE WHEAT PASTA NOODLES (SLIGHTLY BOILED FOR 5MINY.)
1t SEA SALT

SAUTE COLUMNE ONE UNTIL ONIONS ARE LIGHTY BROWN. ADD VEGETABLES IN COLUMN TWO AND SIMMER FOR 10 MIN. THEN ADD COLUMN THREE'S INGREDIENTS STIRRING THEM IN AND ALLOWING TO SIMMER FOR 2-3 MIN AND THEN TURN OFF STOVE. THEN STIRRING IN 1 C OF CASHEW CHEESE SAUCE IS OPTIONAL IN ADDITION.

TOFU STIR FRY

COLUMN ONE	COLUMN TWO
1/2C VEGETABLE OIL	1PACK OF FIRM
1C CHOPPED ONION	TOFU
1C V8 VEGETABLE JUICE	1 ONION SOUP
	PACKAGE
	2 CHOPPED CLOVES OF
	GARLIC
	1T ONION POWDER
	1T GARLIC POWDER
	1t SEA SALT

PRE-SEASON TOFU BY SOAKING IN ONION SOUP POWDER FOR APPRX 20MIN TO 1 HR PRIOR TO SUATING COLUMN ONE . SAUTE COLUMN ONE UNTIL ONIONS ARE LIGHTLY BROWN. THEN ADD SEASONED SLICED TOFU AND ALL REMAINING INGREDIENTS OF COLUMN TWO AND SIMMER FOR 30 MIN THEN TURN OFF STOVE.

OAT BURGERS

COLUMN ONE	COLUMN TWO
6C WATER	1C GROUND
6C LARGE FLAKES OATS	SUNFLOWER SEEDS
3T MOLASSES	
2T SEA SALT	
6 SLICED SMALL ONIONS	
6T GARLIC POWDER	
6T ONION POWDER	
6T BASIL	
6T OREGANO	
1-2t DILL	
2 SLICED WHOLE PEPPERS	
1C NUTRIONAL YEAST FLAKES	

BRING ITEMS IN COLUMN ONE TO A BOIL. ADD ITEMS
OF COLUMN TWO & BRING TO BOIL FOR 5MIN. ALLOW
CONTENTS TO REMAIN IN POT FOR 10MIN TO THICKEN
WHILE STOVE IS TURNED OFF. THEN FORM BURGERS
ON COOKIE SHEET TO BAKE FOR 30 MIN @ 35O F. THEN
TURN THEM OVER FOR 15 MIN THUS COMPLETE.

ALMOND LENTIL LOAF

COLUMN ONE	COLUMN TWO
6C WATER	1C GROUND ALMONDS
3T MOLASSES	
6C LARGE FLAKES OATS	
2T SEA SALT	
2C LENTIL STEW	
6 SLICED SMALL ONIONS	
6T GARLIC POWDER	
6T ONION POWDER	
6T BASIL	
6T OREGANO	
1-2t DILL	
2 SLICED WHOLE PEPPERS	
1C NUTRIONAL YEAST FLAKES	

BRING ITEMS IN COLUMN ONE TO A BOIL. ADD ITEMS OF COLUMN TWO & BRING TO BOIL FOR 5MIN. ALLOW CONTENTS TO REMAIN IN POT FOR 10MIN TO THICKEN WHILE STOVE IS TURNED OFF. THEN PLACE BATTER IN LOAF PAN & BAKE 50-60 MIN (or UNTIL BROWN) @ 350 F.

VEGETABLE POCKET PATTIES

COLUMN ONE	COLUMN TWO
3C PASTA SAUCE	2C WHOLE WHEAT
2T ONION POWDER	FLOUR
1T GARLIC POWDER	1C OAT FLOUR
3C MIXED VEGETABLES	1C WATER
	2T VEGETABLE OIL
	1t SEA SALT

ALLOW COLUMN ONE TO SIMMER FOR 1HR. WHEN THE PASTA SAUCE THICKENS IT IS READY TO USE AS A FILLING. PREPARE DOUGH STIRRING & THEN KNEADING DRY INGREDIENTS INTO WATER. ONCE DOUGH IS FORMED. ROLL DOUGH IN THIN ½ cm FLAT RECTANGLES APPRX 14 cm WIDE (6 inches) & 12 cm LONG (5inches). THEN PLACE 2-3 T OF THICKENED PASTA SAUCE ON RIGHT HALF OF DOUGH. THEN FOLD THE LEFT SIDE OVER MEETING EDGES. THEN ENGRAVE EDGES WITH FORK STICKING EDGES TOGETHER. ONCE PATTIES ARE FORMED THEY MAY BE BAKED FOR 50 MIN @ 350 F IN OVEN. THIS RECIPE MAKES 6-8 PATTIES.

SPREADS

ALMOND MAYONNAISE

BLEND SMOOTH:

1C WATER
1/2C BLANCED RAW ALMONDS
1T ONION POWDER
1T GARLIC POWDER
1t SEA SALT

COOK UNTIL THICK

THEN ADD 1/3C LEMON JUICE

TOFU MAYO

BLEND SMOOTH:

1C WATER
1C TOFU (SOFT & OR FIRM)
1T ONION POWDER
1T GARLIC POWDER
1T HONEY
3T LEMON JUICE
1t SEA SALT

RICE BUTTER

BLEND SMOOTH:

1C COOKED BROWN RICE
¼ C SHREDDED COCONUT
1C WARM WATER
1t SEA SALT

THIS MAY BE SERVED ON BREAD & OR VEGETABLES
AND WILL REMAIN GOOD IN FRIDGE FOR 1 WEEK. THE
RICE MAY BE SUBSTITUTED WITH COOKED MILLET
AS A VARIATION FOR TASTE.

CORN BUTTER

BLEND SMOOTH:

1C COOKED CRISP CORN
3t SHREDDED COCONUT
1C WARM WATER
1t SEA SALT

THIS MAY BE SERVED ON BREAD & OR VEGETABLES
AND WILL REMAIN GOOD IN FRIDGE FOR 1 WEEK.

CASHEW CHEESE

COLUMN ONE

3/4C COOL WATER
1C YEAST FLAKES

1T ONION POWDER
1T GARLIC POWDER
1T SEA SALT
1/3 C PIMENTOS

COLUMN TWO

1 1/4C HOT WATER
2C RINSED RAW
CASHEWS
2T LEMON JUICE

BLEND INGREDIENTS OF COLUMN ONE UNITL CREAMY. ADD COLUMN TWO'S INGREDIENTS AND BLEND UNTIL SMOOTH. CHEESE MAY BE FROZEN FOR UP TO 6 MONTHS.

VEGETABLES ENTREES

STEAMED ASPARAGUS

LAYER:

1 BUNCH OF ASPARAGUS
1/2C OF CASHEW CHEESE SAUCE
1C WATER

CUT ASPARAGUS INTO 3-4 CM PIECES (1-2 INCHES) IN LASAGNE DISH. THEN ADDWATER TO PROVIDE MOISTURE. POUR 1CM (¼ INCH) THICK CREAM CHEESE SAUCE ACROSS ASPARAGUS . THEN COVER DISH & BAKE FOR 10MIN @ 350 F IN MICROWAVE OR 15 MIN IN CONVENTIONAL OVEN.

TASTY BAKED POTATOES

4-6 BAKED POTATOES
1C WATER
2T SEA SALT

WASH POTATOES & DO NOT PEAL SKIN. CUT POTATOES IN HALF & PLACE IN 8X8 PYREX DISH. ADD WATER, THEN SPINKLE SEA SALT LIGHTLY OVER FRESHLY CUT POTATOTES. THEN BAKE IN MICROWAVE FOR 8 MIN OR 30 MIN IN CONVENTIONAL OVEN UNTIL TENDER. THIS WOULD ALLOW FOR A NATURE BUTTERY FLAVOUR TO OCCUR WITH THE BAKED POTATOES WITHOUT THE USE OF BUTTER. YELLOW GOLD POTATOES ARE BEST SUITED FOR THIS RECIPE.

ROASTED SWEET POTATOES

ADD:

6 LARGE SWEET POTATOES
1C VEGETABLE OIL
3T PARSLEY
3T DICED ONION PIECES
1t SEA SALT

CUT SWEET POTATOES IN HALF . DIP POTATES OIL.
APPLY PARSLEY , ONION PIECES & SALT OVER HALVES.
THEN BAKE FOR 50 MIN @ 350 F.

DESSERT ENTREES

BANANA CAKE

MIX:

1C FLEISCHMANN'S NON-HYRDOGENATED
MARGARINE
1 /14C SUGAR (OR SWEETNER OF CHOICE)

THEN ADD & MIX:

1 1/2C SOY/RICE MILK
1-2 RIPE BANANAS
1T VANILLA
1t SEA SALT
1T YEAST
1C WHOLE WHEAT FLOUR
1 1/2C UNBLEACHED WHITE FLOUR

MIX UNTIL BATTER I S SMOOTH AND THICK. THEN
POUR BATTER INTO CAKE /MUFFIN PAN (PRE-
GREASED) & BAKE FOR 50 MIN @ 350 F. A CAKE MIXER IS
AN IDEAL TOOL FOR THIS RECIPE TO ENSURE A SOFT
EVEN TEXTURE IN THE FINAL CAKE PRODUCT.

VANILLA CAKE

MIX:

1C FLEISCHMANN'S NON-HYRDOGENATED
MARGARINE
1 /14C SUGAR (OR SWEETNER OF CHOICE)

THEN ADD & MIX:

1 ½C SOY/RICE MILK
1T VANILLA
1t SEA SALT
1T YEAST
1C WHOLE WHEAT FLOUR
1C UNBLEACHED WHITE FLOUR
¼ C OF CAROB CHIPS & or DRIED FRUIT (OPTIONAL)

MIX UNTIL BATTER IS SMOOTH & THICK (WHICH MAY REQUIRE A SLIGHT ADDITION OF WHITE FLOUR FOR THICKNESS) . THEN POUR BATTER INTO CAKE / MUFFIN PAN (PRE-GREASED) & BAKE FOR 50 MIN @ 350 F. A CAKE MIXER IS AN IDEAL TOOL FOR THIS RECIPE TO ENSURE A SOFT EVEN TEXTURE IN THE FINAL CAKE PRODUCT.

GOD'S PLAN FOR OUR HEALTH

8 LAWS OF HEALTH

NUTRITION: FRUIT, VEGETABLES, GRAINS, LEGUMES AND NUTS

EXERCISE: WALKING IS AN EXCELLENT FORM

WATER: MINIMUM OF 8 GLASSES/DAY OR ENOUGH THAT ALLOWS URINE TO BE PALE IN COLOUR.

SUNSHINE: VITAMIN D IS INTERNTALLY MADE WITH SUNLIGHT EXPOSURE. SUNLIGHT STIMULATES IMMUNIY & MENTAL WELL BEING.

TEMPERENCE: TRUE TEMPERANCE DISPENSES ALL THINGS & OR ACTIVITIES THAT ARE HARMFUL AND USES HEALTHFUL THINGS IN MODERATION.

AIR: SUFFICIENT OXYGEN ALLOWS FOR CLEAR THOUGHT PROCESSESS, REDUCES FATIGUE AND AIDS INTERNAL TOXIN REMOVAL.

REST: REGULAR SLEEP BETWEEN 7-8 HRS BEGINNING 2HRS BEFORE MIDNIGHT IMPROVES SHORT & LONG TERM MEMORY; ALONG WITH AMPLE SECRETION OF GROWTH HORMONE RESPONSIBLE FOR INTERNTAL TISSUE REGENERATION.

TRUST IN GOD: LET THE SOUL BE DRAWN OUT AND UPWARD, THAT GOD MAY GRANT US A BREATH OF THE HEAVENLY ATMOSPHERE. WE MAY KEEP SO NEAR TO GOD THAT IN EVERY UNEXPECTED

TRIAL OUR THOUGHTS WILL TURN TO HIM NATURALLY AS THE FLOWER TO THE SUN. KEEP YOUR WANTS, YOUR JOYS, YOUR SURROWS, YOUR CARES AND YOUR FEARS BEFORE GOD. YOU CANNOT BURDEN HIM YOU CANNOT WEARY HIM. HE WHO NUMBERS THE HAIRS OF YOUR HEAD IS NOT INDIFFERENT TO THE WANTS OF HIS CHILDREN.

CIRCADIAN RHYTHM WITH DIGESTION: CONSUMING A LARGE MEAL FOR BREAKFAST (THE SIZE & PROPROTION OF A NORTH AMERICAN DINNER) WITH A FIVE (5) HOUR INTERVAL OF NO FOOD INTAKE, NOT EVEN A PEANUT OR JUICE. FOLLOWED BY HAVING A LARGE MEAL FOR LUNCH 5HRS LATER AND IF SUPPER

(ANOTHER 5 HRS LATER) CHOOSING FRUIT & OR CEREALS ie. BREAD CRACKERS OR BOXED CEREAL, FOLLOWS THE HORMONAL CHEMISTRY FOR DIGESTION. ONE'S METABOLISM IN RELATION TO DIGESTION IS CHEMICALLY PREPARED TO BEST COVERT FOOD INTO ENERGY AND ABSORB NUTRIENTS BETWEEN THE HOURS OF 5AM- 2PM. THUS ITEMS EASILY DIGESTED SUCH AS FRUIT, VEGETABLES AND OR CEREALS SHOULD PRIMARILY BE TAKEN AT 5-6PM UPON EVENINGS.

GOD'S PLAN FOR OUR HEALTH CONT'D

EXAMPLES OF UNREFINED OR WHOLE GRAINS:

BROWN RICE, WHOLE WHEAT, OATS, RYE, BARLEY, CORN MEAL, BUCKWHEAT, MILLET & QUINOA

BREAKFAST MENU:

FRESH FRUIT, BAKED CEREALS OR FRESH FRUIT AND WHOLE WHEAT BREAD AND OR TOASTED OAT WAFFLES WITH PURE MAPLE SYRUP.

LUNCH MENU:

RICE & PEAS WITH STEWED BEANS, AND SALAD OR TASTY RICE WITH CHICK PEA ALA KING WITH SALAD, OR LASAGNE WITH ROASTED SWEET POTATOES AND SALAD.

THE LORD HAS PROMISED III JOHN 3:2; BELOVED, I WISH ABOVE ALL THINGS THAT THOU MAYEST PROSPER AND BE IN HEALTH EVEN AS THY SOUL PROSPERETH.

MAY THIS BE YOUR EXPERIENCE BY GOD'S GRACE.

CORONARY ARTERY DISEASE

Coronary Artery Disease also known as Heart Disease is one of the leading causes of death in Canada. It may be defined as progressive damage to blood vessels due to arteriosclerosis also known as hardening of the arteries. Arteries become damaged by continual deposits of excess cholesterol, calcium and platelets floating in the blood circulation. These are deposited within the muscular layer of blood vessels. Thus blood vessels loose elasticity over time, become completely occluded and or erupt preventing needed blood circulation to the heart muscle or the brain. Hence Coronary Artery disease leads to Cardiac Arrests (Heart Attacks) or Strokes (Cerebral Vascular Disease).

It has been estimated that over one third of all deaths in Canada are due to Coronary Artery Disease. Approximately 80.2% of all Canadians age 20-50 years of age have at least one contributing risk factor of Heart disease costing health care an estimated $19 million annually.

The signs and symptom typical with Coronary Artery Disease include High Blood Pressure (Hypertension, Irregular Heart beats, Angina commonly known as Chest pain, and Increasing fatigue with activity or exertion. The initial and most typical warning sign is an elevated High Blood pressure which can go unnoticed for years as usually painless.

Risk factors known to directly contribute to Coronary Artery Disease, include a diet especially high in cholesterol and then saturated fats. Other risk factors include, smoking, sedentary life styles, Diabetes, Obesity and Stress. Though high salt intake may raise blood pressures it is not the direct contributing cause to Heart Disease rather, elevated cholesterol levels are. It has been confirmed that North Americans by age 15 have noted cholesterol streaks already deposited in blood vessels potentially leading to their hardening.

The good news about Coronary Artery Disease is that it may be prevented, reversed and or improved with good management depending as to how early and consistently changes are made. It is very important that regular blood pressure assessments are done to ascertain patterns. If Hypertensive or diagnosed with Coronary Artery Disease it is best to eliminate dietary cholesterol and lower saturated fats. Increase foods that contain Fibre ie. Fruit, Vegetables, Whole grains and Legumes. Fibre removes cholesterol that is either stored in Blood vessels and accumulated in the Intestinal tract. Exercise is also important to elevate good cholesterol levels. However increased exercise must be coupled with dietary changes. These changes should be done in partnership with your doctor who can determine which medications may be needed depending upon how advanced the disease is or improved with changes suggested. The final analysis is improved longevity and quality of life for your well being.

DIABETES MELLITUS

Diabetes Mellitus is the disease process in which Insulin resistance develops over time. Its development occurs as the receptor sites on cells no longer correspond with Insulin attempting to bring glucose into cellular activity. Normal Blood Glucose should range from 4-6 mmol/L. It is important to have one's Blood sugar tested regularly , the most accurate being the Glycosylated Hemoglobin Test.

There are two main types of the Disease that will be addressed. Insulin dependent Diabetes known as Type I or IDDM occurs between ages 2-21 years of age. This form is also known as Juvenile-onset Diabetes. Type I occurs when the Pancreas is unable to produce Insulin. Non-Insulin-Dependent or Type II Diabetes is also known as the Adult onset form of this disease. Unfortunately, due to increasing numbers of childhood Obesity, Type II Diabetes is more increasingly being diagnosed in children and teenagers rather than in adults 40-50 years of age during the past 10 years. With this form of Diabetes the Pancreas produces Insulin; however the receptor sites are less responsive to this (Insulin) hormone. The result then is the inability to transfer glucose into cells. In an effort to compensate the Pancreas will over produce Insulin. This reaction stimulates the production of excess of cholesterol and future Coronary Artery Disease. Risk factors that predispose individuals to Type I disease, include viral infections or a Genetic predisposition to Dairy allergies, which could contribute to Beta cell destruction in the Pancreas responsible for Insulin production. Risk factors for Type II include Obesity, High Saturated & or Cholesterol Fat, and a Sedentary Lifestyle.

Clinical Manifestations present in both Type I and Type II Diabetes, include Fatigue, Dizziness, Excessive hunger or thirst, frequent urination at night, and most serious, a Coma. Individuals with the Type I form of the disease may more rapidly develop a coma if blood sugars are not well managed. The critical side effects of either Types of Diabetes include Glaucoma, Blindness, Neuropathy (Nerve damage), Peripheral Vascular disease, Coronary Artery Disease and Kidney Disease.

The best management of either Type of Diabetes should include a High Complex Carbohydrate (Fibre) Diet, which reduces the rate in which Glucose is absorbed from the Small Intestinal tract into the Blood Circulation. Reduction of High Fat intake and Regular Exercise contributes to weight loss or management and improves the Insulin cellular receptor site response thus lowering high blood sugars. For Type I Diabetes this pattern could lead to the reduction of Insulin units needed. Type II Diabetics on this program would less likely deteriorate with the need of transferring from hypoglycemic medications to Insulin. Rather Hypoglycemic mediations could be reduced, to the point where Blood Sugars could be managed by Lifestyle alone. As a Consultant, I have noted much in improvement in Blood sugars with these interventions.

This program should be done in collaboration with One's Doctor. The end result, being the best quality of health in Diabetic Health management.

ENERGIZING THE NERVOUS SYSTEM

The Nervous System is comprised of approximately 100 billion neurons. Neurons are nerve cells that conduct electrical impulses which are messages that result in changes in mobility and organ secretions. This system is divided into two major categories being the Central and Peripheral Nervous System.

The Central Nervous System (CNS system) is comprised of the Brain and the Spinal cord. Together they coordinate messages for many essential activities in the Human body that include the process of thinking, speaking, breathing and mobility. Nerve conduction is this system either Collect, Transmit Analyze and or Send information to allow for the best response to a situation or stimulus.

The Peripheral Nervous System is responsible for the transfer of information branching from the Central Nervous System to smooth muscles and or organs. It is subdivided into the Sensory and Motor Nervous System. The Sensory Nervous System conducts messages to internal organs as influenced from external stimuli to the body.

The Motor Nervous System conducts messages that manage smooth, skeletal and the cardiac (heart) muscles.

The Motor Nervous System is further subdivided into the Somatic and Autonomic systems. The Somatic Nervous System manage nerve impulses that control the movement of Skeletal muscles such as arms, legs and those found in skin. The Autonomic system manages nerve impulses that convey information which manages smooth and or the cardiac muscle.

The ability of the Central nervous system to enhance mental concentration, improve memory and emotional well being is dependent upon a few factors. One includes the amount of B complex vitamins that are available in dietary intake. Vitamin B complex vitamins such as Thiamin and or Riboflavin improve nerve conduction even in the Cerebral (frontal) lobe of the Brain. The increased hours of sleep prior to midnight improves Short term memory which subsequently strengthens the transfer of information into Long Term memory. This then improves coordination and precision with complex details managed during the day. The use of caffeine reduces the availability Phosphodiesterase (PDE) an important enzyme system needed for memory development. Caffeine also disrupts Neurotransmitters such as Acetylcholine, Adenosine and Dopamine which can increase Insomnia, Anxiety and Depression and inaccurate work performance. Melatonin is a hormone that stimulates Cerebral nerve endings to improve cognitive and emotional well being. It is designed in the Pineal Gland and stored in the Pituitary gland of the brain. It is found in high quantities in food sources such as rice and corn. Finally a High Complex Carbohydrate (fibre) diet low in saturated and cholesterol fats, reduces fat accumulation in tiny Blood vessels that support the Cerebral Nerve conduction.

STRENGHTHENING
THE IMMUNE SYSTEM

Immunity is the process in which the human body protects itself from becoming infected and or destroyed by microbes. Microbes are cellular bodies that invade and destroy normal human cells such as bacteria, fungi, parasites or viruses. The Integumentary system being the human skin matrix is one of the initial barriers to such invaders. The PH level of saliva, coupled with Hydrochloric acid which is secreted into the stomach during digestion are capable of destroying significant populations of microbes before replicating in the intestinal region. Repetitive deep breathing that occurs with regular exercise increases the concentration of Oxygen that can denature the presence of anaerobic bacteria that cannot survive in this gas.

Microbes escaping these initial phases of immunity tend to invade rapidly during prolonged periods of negative stressors, fatigue and chilling of the extremities. It is then White Blood Cell activity becomes the significant component for immunity.

Differing types of White Blood Cells have specific roles in providing immunity. One, Macrophages consumes bacteria and when overwhelmed release lymphokine secretions (chemical messengers) to call aid from Helper T cells. Helper T cells are informed by Macrophages the type of microbe invader and will send additional lymphokine to request aid from either Killer T cells that secrete enzymes to destroy microbes and carcinogens and or B lymph cells that form antibodies to destroy bacteria specifically. Suppressor B & T cells are then summoned to end the entire immune response when the microbes are destroyed. Followed, by Memory T and or B cells that make genetic memory files to better aid the war against the identical microbe invading the body again. Chemical toxins that are environmental or are byproducts of digestion are also denatured by the immune system.

The strength of the immune system is dependent upon how many hours of sleep the body receives prior to midnight. The degree to which immunity is invigorated through exercise. The presence of cholesterol and excess sugar in the blood stream greatly reduces the speed and defensive nature of White Blood Cell activity. Dairy products contain significant amounts of cholesterol. Normal Blood PH is said to be between 7.35-7.45 with the latter to be known as slightly alkaline. PH readings closer to 7.45, have been noted to inhibit the ability of microbe reproduction hence also aiding the immunity against infectious disease. A diet high in fruit, vegetables and whole grains results in normal alkaline PH levels of 7.4. Hence a Life Style that consists of a High fiber, Low fat diet with good exercise and rest, are key determinants to ensuring improved and strengthened immunity.

NUTRITION INFORMATION

Vitamin B 1 –Thiamin:

> Found in Whole wheat, Oats,
> Barley , Brown Rice, Corn, Whole
> Grain Rye, Beans, Peas, Nuts

Vitamin B 2 Riboflavin:

> Found in Whole wheat, Oats,
> Barley , Brown Rice, Corn, Whole
> Grain Rye, Beans, Peas, Nuts

Vitamin B 3 Niacin:

> Found in Whole wheat, Oats,
> Barley , Brown Rice, Corn, Whole
> Grain Rye, Beans, Peas, Nuts

Vitamin B 5 Pantothenic:

> Found in Whole wheat, Oats,
> Barley , Brown Rice, Corn, Whole
> Grain Rye, Beans, Peas, Nuts

Vitamin B 6 Pyridoxine:

> Found in Whole wheat, Oats,
> Barley , Brown Rice, Corn, Whole
> Grain Rye, Beans, Peas, Nuts

Vitamin B12 Cobalamin:

> Found in Whole Wheat

Minerals

Calcium:

Oats, Beans, Nuts , Broccoli,
Collards, Kale, Molasses, Sesame Seeds

Iron:

Oats, Lentils, Lima Beans, Pigeon Peas,
Chick Peas, Beets, Molasses,
Dried Apricots,

Antioxidants

Vitamin A Beta-carotene :

Red, Green and Yellow Fruit &
Vegetables

Vitamin E Alpha- tocopherol & Gama-tocopherol:

Asparagus, Avocados, Nuts, Seeds
& Whole Wheat

Vitamin C:

Raw Fruit and Vegetables

Resveratrol:

Red Grapes

Lutein:

        Spinach

Isoflavines:

        Soy

Proanthocyanidins:

        Berries

BIBLIOGRAPHY

Batmanghelidj, F. MD. 1997. *Your Body's Many Cries For Water.* Virginia: Global Health Solutions Inc.

http://www.crumcreek.com/library/antioxidant.html

Foster, Vernon W. MD. 1990. *New Start.* California. Vernon Foster.

Howell, Edward Dr. 1985. *Enzyme nutrition: The Food Enzyme Concept.* New Jersey Avery Publishing Group Inc.

Jaret, Peter. 1986. *Our Immune System: The Wars With.* National Geographic.

Lee, Celeste. 1992. *Understanding The Body Organs & The Eight Laws of Health.* New York: Teach Series.

Lee, Deborah. 1997. *Essential Fatty Acids.* Woodland Publishing Inc. The Woodland Health Series.

Lewis, Sharon M. & Collier, Idolia C. 1987. *Medical-Surgical Nursing: Assessment And Management of Clinical Problems.* New York: McGraw-Hill Book Company.

Nedley, Neil MD. 1999. Proof Positive: How to Reliably Combat Disease and Achieve Optimal Health through Nutrition and Lifestyle. NW, Ardmore, OK: Neil Nedley.

Nedley, Neil MD. 2001. *Depression: The Way Out.* NW, Ardmore, OK: Neil Nedley.

Roehl, Evelyn. 1996. Whole Food Facts: The Complete Reference Guide. Vermount Healing Arts Press.

Thrash, Agatha & Calvin MDs. 1981. *Homes Remedies: Hydrotherapy, Massage, Charcoal and Other Simple Treatments*. Alabama: Thrash Publications.

Thrash, Agatha & Calvin MDs. 1996. *Nutrition for Vegetarians*. Alabama: Thrash Publications.